Diabetes Mastery

The Game-Changing Method for Overcoming Insulin Resistance in All Diabetes Forms (Type 1, Type 1.5, Type 2, Prediabetes, and Gestational Diabetes) and Take Control of Your Health

By

Mark R. Dickson

Disclaimer

Copyright © by Mark R. Dickson 2024.
All rights reserved.

Table of Contents

Appendix

Introduction

People who are living with diabetes have a broad variety of options available to them when it comes to dealing with things like glucose and food.

There are some people who adhere to low-carb or ketogenic diets and consume fewer carbohydrates, some like tracking calories with more adjusted macronutrients, and yet others are dieters who a vegetable enthusiasts to the extreme.

Although these eating plans are effective, we do not advocate for a single dietary approach that is particularly nourishing here on Diabetes Solid. After taking everything into consideration, we are of the opinion that you ought to be aware of the numerous options available to you so that you may make an informed decision regarding what is suitable for you, your body, and your diabetes.

As part of our discussion today, we will look into the incredibly unique plant-based, high-carb method that is described in the book The Diabetes Code for Space.

In recent times, I have had the privilege of exploring the Dominating Diabetes method of addressing the issue of sustenance for those who are dealing with diabetes.

This is captivating. In spite of the fact that it is completely dissimilar to the way in which I live my life, it can very well be the most suitable option for you.
When you are living with diabetes, you might want to think about how to make a high-carb diet work for you, or you might want to examine why this would be something possible. To react to a fraction of these queries, I plunked down with Robby Barbaro to analyze the new book and become familiar with a bit more about the Dominating Diabetes strategy and the manner of thinking that drives it.

Chapter 1: What is Diabetes Mystery Method and how does it work?

The Dominating Diabetes Technique is a framework that is meant to invert insulin antagonism. To begin with, we should audit what insulin blockage is and why it's something that would surely value learning.

Insulin resistance develops when your muscles and liver have an impaired reaction to the activity of insulin. This is brought about by the storage of an overabundance of fat in tissues that are not intended to retain vast amounts of fat, bringing about a diminished capacity of insulin to advance glucose take-up in both muscle and liver cells.

Insulin opposition influences individuals living with all types of diabetes (counting type 1, type 1.5, prediabetes, type 2, and gestational diabetes), which decisively builds your gamble for coronary supply route sickness, atherosclerosis, malignant growth, elevated cholesterol, hypertension, stoutness, fringe neuropathy, retinopathy, Alzheimer's infection, chronic renal disease, and greasy liver illness.

How does this method switch insulin obstruction?

Our technique switches insulin obstruction by supporting you with lowering how much surplus fat has formed in your muscle and liver cells. Those phones can then get back to putting away a proper proportion of fat.

This is achieved by:

*Low-fat, plant-based, entire food sustenance: We propose eating food sources that are generally low in fat, and rich in fiber, water, and supplement thickness to emphatically further increase your insulin response. These food kinds combine organic items, bland veggies, vegetables, undamaged entire grains, non-boring vegetables, mixed greens, spices, tastes, and mushrooms.

- Irregular Fasting: Changing the planning of your food admittance is one of the most remarkable strategies for further increasing your insulin awareness, working on your cardiovascular well-being, and getting thinner. Dominating Diabetes demonstrates you how to plan and adopt a supportable irregular fasting habit to change your metabolic well-being.

- Everyday Development: Your body is intended for actual work, and when you make day-to-day development a component of your way of life, you're probably going to emphatically further develop your insulin responsiveness, energy levels, and temperament.

How would you deal with blood glucose increases on a high-carb diet?

For persons living with insulin-subordinate diabetes, there are a handful of keys to forestalling post-feast blood glucose spikes:

- Put up a tremendous effort to guarantee that your fat admittance doesn't beyond 30 grams each day (or a limit of 15% of entire calories)

- Eat a full sugar-rich meal that is loaded with water, fiber, nutrients, minerals, cell reinforcements, and phytochemicals

- Progress to a plant-based diet gradually across 1-2 months, and emphasis on modifying just a single dinner at a time. This permits you to roll out little changes to your insulin or maybe pharmaceutical methods and supports you with understanding what every feast entails for your blood glucose control.

- Focus on insulin timing and ensuring your blood glucose is 120 mg/dL and moving down before eating a sugar-rich dinner (utilizing a fingerstick blood glucose measurement).

- For those living with non-insulin subservient diabetes, use the Dominating Diabetes Strategy the precise method we illustrate in the book by assessing your degree of benchmark insulin opposition.

- For those with a greater degree of benchmark insulin blockage, we propose using a 2-step technique by eating low-glycemic food sources for the initial not many weeks followed by higher-glycemic food sources throughout time. This permits you to mix extra vegetables into your eating regimen while lowering the chance of hyperglycemia.

Could you at any point follow the Dominating Diabetes Strategy effectively in the event that you're not vegetarian?

Indeed, totally. We have a traffic signal food structure with a green light, yellow light, and red light food variations in which we recommend you to eat an eating routine incorporating whatever a number of plant food types as could be expected under the circumstances.
In the event that you decide not to consume a 100 percent plant-based diet, you can in any case eat modest quantities of creature products found in the red light class and start switching insulin blockage typically.

Truly we are not the food police. We basically recommend you to consume an eating routine including whatever number of plants as could be expected under the conditions to improve your insulin responsiveness, be that as it may, your craving to limit or kill creature items is fully up to your individual selection.

Are there any downsides or anything one ought to be aware of?

The worst downside is that you'll be able to simply limit your usage of delectable high-fat food kinds like avocados, nuts, seeds, and coconut meat to enhance your insulin awareness genuinely

Know about the quantity of the food kinds you are devouring to ensure your improvement is essentially as smooth as could be predicted. A minimal quantity is useful, although it's remarkably simple to indulge in greasy food items, which adversely affect blood glucose regulation.

Chapter 2: The Difference Between Insulin Resistance and Diabetes?

Anybody can acquire insulin resistance — for a little time or consistently. Over the long haul, persistent insulin obstruction can motivate prediabetes and afterward Type 2 diabetes on the off chance that it's not managed or ready to be dealt with.

Prediabetes develops when your blood glucose levels are greater than typical, but not sufficiently high to be assessed as diabetes. Prediabetes normally arises in persons who as of now have some insulin opposition.

Prediabetes can prompt Sort 2 diabetes (T2D), the most well-known kind of diabetes. T2D develops when your pancreas doesn't create sufficient insulin or your body doesn't utilize insulin well (insulin opposition), bringing in high blood glucose levels.

Type 1 diabetes (T1D) develops when your body's safe framework assaults and obliterates the insulin-creating cells in your pancreas for an unknown explanation. T1D is an immune system and continuing ailment, and individuals with T1D need to infuse tailored insulin to live and be sound. While T1D isn't brought about by insulin obstruction, persons with T1D can face levels of insulin opposition in which their cells don't respond properly to the insulin they infuse.

Gestational diabetes is a short kind of diabetes that can occur during pregnancy. It's created by insulin blockage that is expected from the substances the placenta generates. Gestational diabetes vanishes once you convey your child. Roughly 3% to 8% of people who are pregnant individuals in the US are determined to have gestational diabetes.

Medical care suppliers typically apply a blood test called glycated hemoglobin (A1c) to assess diabetes. It indicates your normal glucose level over the past 90 days. Overall:

An A1c level below 5.7% is seen as usual.

An A1c reading anywhere in the range of 5.7% and 6.4% is called prediabetes.

An A1c reading of 6.5% or greater on two independent tests reveals type 2 diabetes.

Individuals with Type 1 diabetes normally have an incredibly high A1C and extremely high blood glucose levels upon finding it in view of the fact that their pancreas is supplying very little or no insulin.

What are the signs of insulin obstruction?

Assuming you have insulin obstruction, nevertheless, your pancreas can boost insulin manufacturing to keep your glucose levels in range, and you will not have any negative effects.

Notwithstanding, after some time, insulin blockage can deteriorate, and the cells in your pancreas that make insulin can break down. Ultimately, your pancreas is as of now not equipped to generate sufficient insulin to beat the opposition, leading to elevated glucose (hyperglycemia), which causes negative effects.

Symptoms of elevated glucose include:

- Expanded thirst.
- Regular urine (peeing).
- Expanded hunger.
- Obscured vision.
- Cerebral aches.
- Vaginal and cutaneous contaminations.
- Slow-mending cuts and bruises.

Many individuals have no side symptoms of prediabetes, frequently for quite a long time. Prediabetes could be unnoticeable until it evolves into Type 2 diabetes. Certain persons with prediabetes may suffer the accompanying adverse effects:

Obscured skin in your armpit or back and sides of your neck, called acanthosis nigricans.

Skin labels (little skin developments).

Eye alterations can induce diabetes-related retinopathy.

On the off chance that you're confronting any of these negative effects, seeing your medical care provider is significant.

What causes insulin opposition?

Researchers actually have a ton to discover about how precisely insulin blockage produces. Up to this moment, they've distinguished a few traits that make an individual quite substantially susceptible to fostering insulin opposition. Furthermore, more established persons are more likely to have insulin blockage.

A few variables and circumstances can produce varying levels of insulin opposition. Researchers acknowledge that overabundance of muscle-to-fat ratio, notably around your abdomen, and genuine inertia are the two major contributing parts to insulin opposition.

Gained explanations for insulin blockage Obtained causes, the importance you're not brought into the world with the reason, of insulin blockage include:

*** Overabundance muscle fat ratio**: Researchers believe corpulence, specifically overabundance of fat in your belly and around your organs (instinctive fat), is an important driver of insulin obstruction. A midsection estimation of 40 inches or anything else for guys and individuals doled out male upon entering the world and 35 inches or whatever else for ladies and people demoted to female upon entering the world is associated with insulin opposition. Studies have demonstrated that stomach fat releases chemicals and other compounds that can add to long-haul aggravation in your body. This irritation can assume a part in insulin opposition

* **Actual idleness**: Active work makes your body more delicate to insulin and creates muscle that can retain blood glucose. An absence of genuine employment can produce inverse impacts and cause insulin blockage. Likewise, an absence of vigorous work and an inactive way of life are associated with weight growth, which can likewise lead to insulin opposition.

* **Diet:** An eating regimen of profoundly handled, high-sugar food kinds and soaking fats has been associated with insulin opposition. Your body processes extremely handled, high-carb food variety fast, which causes your glucose to jump. This puts additional weight on your pancreas to release a ton of insulin, which, over the long run, can cause insulin opposition.

* **Certain prescriptions**: Certain drugs can induce insulin blockage, including steroids, some pulse meds, certain HIV medicines, and a few psychiatric pills.

How is insulin blockage treated?

Since not all circumstances that add to insulin obstruction can be dealt with, for example, hereditary factors and age, way-of-life alterations are the fundamental remedy for insulin opposition. Way of life changes include:

* **Eating a sound eating regimen**: Your medical services provider or nutritionist might propose trying not to consume inordinate measures of carbs (which quickens the overabundance of insulin manufacture) and eating less unwanted fat, sugar, red meats, and handled starches. All things being equal, they'll usually advocate eating an eating regimen of entire food sources that combines more veggies, organic items, entire grains, fish, and lean poultry.

* **Actual work:** Getting customary measures of moderate-power physical labor assists in enhancing glucose energy utilization and further

developing muscle insulin awareness. A solitary meeting of moderate-power exercise can augment glucose take-up by no less than 40%.

* **Losing abundant weight**: Your medical services supplier can advise attempting to lose overabundance weight to take a stab at treating insulin opposition. One study found that decreasing 7% of your excess weight can reduce the beginning of Type 2 diabetes by 58%.

After some time, this way of life modifications can:

- Increment insulin responsiveness (diminish insulin blockage).
- Bring a decrease in your blood glucose levels.
- Decline circulatory strain.
- Decline fatty substance and LDL ("terrible") cholesterol levels.
- Raise HDL ("great") cholesterol levels.

You might collaborate with other medical services suppliers, for example, a nutritionist and endocrinologist, notwithstanding your typical specialist to conceive of a unique therapy approach that turns out the finest for you.

What medicines are utilized to treat insulin obstruction?

While there are right now no prescriptions that address insulin obstruction directly, your medical services supplier might propose drugs to treat coinciding conditions. A few models include:

- Pulse prescription.
- Metformin for diabetes.
- Statins to bring down LDL cholesterol.

Chapter 3: All Fats Are Not Made Equally

There is a great deal of contradicting data out there about fats and on the off chance that there is a strategy for integrating them into your eating regimen in a sensible manner. Fortunately, dietary fats are a crucial aspect of a balanced eating regimen, and not all fats are manufactured identical.

With regards to fats, the major purpose is to substitute food supplies rich in soaking fats (greasy portions of meat, chicken with skin, high-fat dairy items like cream, spread, and complete milk, coconut oil, and other tropical oils) with food sources wealthy in unsaturated fats.

Endeavor to merge additional monounsaturated and polyunsaturated fats into your dietary regimen instead of immersed fats to assist with decreasing your aggregate and "awful" LDL cholesterol.

Monounsaturated fats aid in augmenting the "upside" cholesterol in the body known as HDL cholesterol. At the point when you pick these fats you can reduce the danger of generating a cardiovascular sickness. Instances of food types abundant in monounsaturated fats include:

- Avocados
- Pumpkin seeds and sesame seeds are two examples of seeds.
- Nuts and nut spreads such as almonds, almond margarine, peanuts, peanut butter, and walnuts
- Olives
- Vegetable oils, for example, canola oil, olive oil, and nut oil

Polyunsaturated fats are a wellspring of essential omega-3 and omega-6 fats that are not produced by the body and in this way should be gained from food sources. Omega-3 fats especially can assist with improving cardiac well-being by diminishing fatty oils (a kind of fat in the blood); easing back the development of plaque in the courses, and decreasing irritation in the body. Polyunsaturated fats are tracked down in a vast range of food sorts, including:

- Fish like fish, salmon, mackerel, and trout
- Flaxseeds, chia seeds, hemp seeds, pumpkin seeds, and sunflower seeds
- Vegetable oils, for example, corn oil, sunflower oil, and soybean oil
- Pecans

The following are a handful of basic strategies for integrating more heart-sound fats into your food routine:

- Top your oats or cold oats with a small bunch of nuts or almonds for some added crunch.
- Trade out locally purchased, mayo-based dressing and prepare your own dish of

mixed greens dressing with olive oil, balsamic vinegar, lemon juice, new garlic, and dark pepper.

- Attempt to recall fish high for omega-3 fats in your feasts no less than two times each week.
- Two or three cuts of avocado to your sandwich rather than mayonnaise or margarine.
- Add flaxseeds, chia seeds, or hemp seeds to your oats to give them a substantially creamier surface.
- Cook or prepare with canola oil or other plant-based oils rather than margarine.
- Eliminate the skin from chicken and turkey.
- Add unsalted sunflower or pumpkin seeds to your dish of mixed greens for a decent crunch.

These goods are accessible in nearly all supermarkets, so anytime you're buying, make certain to add them to your truck. Then, at that point, have some good times investigating alternative pathways regarding ways of integrating them into your eating regimen. Your heart will be much obliged.

Virginia Heart is Northern Virginia's leading cardiovascular gathering, with in excess of 50 board-guaranteed cardiologists who give expertise in treating different situations that influence the body's heart and vascular frameworks.

Chapter 4: What Are Carbohydrates?

Carbs are the sugars and starches tracked down in diet. There are two essential forms of carbs: complex and basic. Complex sugars exist in grains, vegetables, and some plants — like potatoes and corn. Organic food, dairy items, and pastries for the most part contain plain sugars. Refined starches are likewise a form of basic carb, with a huge number of the normal fixings and supplements removed. A few instances of refined carbs involve soft drinks, white flour goods, and high-fructose corn syrup.

So now let's break it down!!!

Carbohydrates: The Fuel for Your Body

Carbohydrates - they're more than just a dietary buzzword; they're the powerhouse behind the energy that propels us through our daily lives. But what exactly are carbohydrates, and why do they play such a pivotal role in our overall well-being?

In the simplest terms, carbohydrates are one of the three essential macronutrients, alongside proteins and fats. These compounds, composed of carbon, hydrogen, and oxygen, are the primary source of energy for the human body. From the slice of toast you savor in the morning to the pasta that fills your dinner plate, carbohydrates are omnipresent in our diets.

Types of Carbohydrates: The Good, the Bad, and the Complex

Not all carbohydrates are created equal. They come in various forms, and understanding these distinctions is key to making informed dietary choices.

Simple Carbohydrates: Imagine these as the Usain Bolts of the carbohydrate world - quick to break down and provide a burst of energy. Found in sugary treats, fruits, and refined grains, simple carbohydrates can offer a rapid energy boost. However, their effects are often short-lived, leading to the infamous sugar crash that leaves you reaching for another energy fix sooner rather than later.

Complex Carbohydrates: Picture these as the marathon runners, pacing themselves for the long haul. Complex carbohydrates, found in whole grains, legumes, and vegetables, take more time to digest. This gradual breakdown ensures a sustained release of energy, keeping you fueled throughout the day without the rollercoaster of sugar highs and lows.

The Glorious Role of Carbohydrates in Your Body

Carbohydrates are not just about energizing your next workout; they're the VIPs supporting various bodily functions. When you consume carbohydrates, your body breaks them down into glucose, a form of sugar that serves as the primary fuel for your brain and muscles.

Ever wondered why athletes load up on carbs before a big race? It's not just a tradition; it's a science-backed strategy. Carbohydrate stores, mainly in the form of glycogen in muscles and the liver, act as a readily available energy reservoir during strenuous activities. So, that pre-race pasta dinner is like topping off your body's gas tank for optimal performance.

Carbs and Blood Sugar

The relationship between carbohydrates and blood sugar is a delicate dance. When you consume carbohydrates, your body converts them into glucose, causing blood sugar levels to rise. In response, the pancreas releases insulin, a hormone that facilitates the absorption of glucose by cells for energy.

However, not all carbs are equal when it comes to blood sugar impact. Simple carbohydrates, like those in candies and sodas, can lead to rapid spikes, prompting a swift insulin response. This rollercoaster can contribute to insulin resistance over time, a precursor to diabetes.

On the flip side, complex carbohydrates offer a more gradual and steady release of glucose, allowing the body to manage blood sugar levels more effectively. Choosing whole, unprocessed foods over refined options becomes a strategy for maintaining a balanced and sustainable blood sugar profile.

The Carb Conundrum: Finding Your Balance

In a world bombarded by low-carb diets and carbophobia, it's essential to remember that not all carbohydrates are the enemy. Rather than demonizing an entire macronutrient, the key lies in making informed choices.

Balancing your carbohydrate intake with a mix of whole grains, fruits, vegetables, and legumes ensures you receive the benefits of sustained energy without the drawbacks of excessive sugar consumption. It's not about forsaking carbs but embracing the right kind in the right amounts.

3 Motivations to Lower Your Carbohydrates Intakes

Starches are not especially horrible. They are the least challenging sort of energy that our bodies can process. Nonetheless, there are several motives to direct your carb consumption, including:

1. To manage insulin levels. Carbs – simply basic carbs — might make your insulin levels glucose levels surge not long after you eat them. Not in the least does this lead you to feel drowsy, however, it can prompt insulin opposition and boost your chance for type 2 diabetes.

2. To better develop energy. The uncomplicated sub-atomic design of carbs indicates your body makes them into speedy, basic energy that you consume rapidly. This can lead you to feel more tired or hungry over the course of the day. Reducing your sugar consumption and consuming more protein and solid fats provides your body greater admission to progressively moving energy sources.

3. To augment supplements. Refined starches are robbed of their fiber and vitamins so your body can absorb them rapidly. Complex carbs supply additional fiber and minerals per serving, so you ought to likewise ingest these with some limitations. Set aside a lot of space for protein, nutrient-stuffed veggies, and fiber-filled food choices in your eating routine by avoiding carbs. This will lead you to feel more full for longer since you're offering your body sufficient amounts of nutrients and supplements.

While low-carb diets will aid you with reducing your sugar consumption, you ought to constantly consult with a dietician, nutritionist, or one more experienced clinical expert while contemplating any big alterations to your meal plan.

Chapter 5: Diagnostics Blood Tests and Managing Oral Medications

How Are Diabetes and Prediabetes Diagnosed?

The accompanying tests are utilized for the conclusion of diabetes:

A fasting plasma glucose test assesses your blood glucose after you have gone something like 8 hours without eating. This test is performed to recognize diabetes or prediabetes.
An oral glucose resilience test assesses your glucose after you have gone no less than eight hours without eating and two hours after you drink a glucose-containing refreshment. This test can be applied to examine diabetes or prediabetes.
In an irregular plasma glucose test, your PCP tests your glucose regardless of when you ate

your last dinner. This test, alongside an assessment of side effects, is utilized to examine diabetes, nevertheless not prediabetes.

A hemoglobin A1c (HbA1c) test should be possible without fasting and can be employed to examine or verify either prediabetes or diabetes.

Positive trial results ought to be affirmed by rehashing the fasting plasma glucose test or the oral glucose resilience test on an alternative day. At the point when initially found to have diabetes, your PCP could recommend a zinc carrier 8 autoantibodies (ZnT8Ab) test. This blood test - - plus other data and trial outcomes - - can assist in identifying whether an individual has type 1 diabetes and not another form. The purpose of having the ZnT8Ab test is a brief and exact assessment that can prompt easy treatment.

Fasting Plasma Glucose (FPG) Test
The FPG is most dependable when done at the beginning of the day. Assuming your fasting glucose level is 100 to 125 mg/dL, you have a

type of prediabetes termed weakened fasting glucose (IFG), meaning that you are bound to foster sort 2 diabetes yet don't have it yet. A degree of 126 mg/dL or higher, affirmed by repeating the test on one more day, suggests that you have diabetes.

Do I Want an Oral Glucose Resistance Test?

Your glucose level can give your primary care physician substantial suggestions about your well-being, and an oral glucose resistance test (OGTT) demonstrates how effectively your body manages sugar from dietary choices.

It can figure out if you are in danger of diabetes or then again in the event that you as of now have it. A more limited depiction of an OGTT examines for diabetes during pregnancy.
Regularly when you eat, your glucose rises. Your pancreas, a lengthy organ somewhere down in the midsection, delivers a hormone called insulin. It assists movement with sugaring from your blood into your phones for energy and

capacity. Then, at that point, your glucose returns to usual.

Assuming that you have type 2 diabetes, your body utilizes insulin insufficiently. Glucose develops in your blood. This overload of sugar might injure the veins throughout your body. Diabetes might cause coronary disease, neurological injury, eye sickness, and kidney harm.

When Do I Need the Test?

You could require an oral glucose resilience test on the off chance that you:

- Are overweight or obese
- Have a neighboring relative with diabetes
- Have hypertension
- Have excessive fatty compounds (a form of fat in your blood)
- Have polycystic ovarian dysfunction (which generates feminine difficulties)

- Conveyed an infant who weighed in excess of 9 pounds
- Had gestational diabetes during a former pregnancy
- A more limited form of this test is finished between the 24th and 28th seven-day stretch of pregnancy to check whether you have gestational diabetes. It's known as the oral glucose challenge test.

How Would I Prepare?

To arrive at an exact outcome on the OGTT, eat roughly 150 grams of carbs every day for 3 days before the test. Try not to eat or drink anything with the exception of water after roughly 10 o'clock the prior night.

You don't have to conduct any unique prep before the pregnancy glucose challenge test. Simply remain away from food choices containing a great deal of sugar, like doughnuts or squeezed oranges.

How Is It Done?

You'll get the OGTT at your PCP's office, a center, a clinic, or a lab. This occurs:

- A medical caretaker or specialist will take a blood test from a vein in your arm to test your initial glucose level.
- You'll next, at that point, consume a combination of glucose disintegrated in water.
- You'll get another blood glucose test 2 hours after the fact.
- During pregnancy, the test is more limited. You'll drink a delicious fluid. Then, at that point, you'll have a blood test roughly one hour after the incident.

Chapter 6: How Profound Breathing Might Assist in Controlling Glucose, Further Developing Wellbeing

Profound breathing accompanies heaps of advantages from regulating glucose levels to further improving lung capability.

Stress can influence your invulnerability and your risk of diabetes, heart disease, and malignant development also goes up when you experience consistent pressure.

Stress can negatively influence your well-being. It weakens existing medical troubles as well as endangers you or several individuals. To put it clearly, in the event that you are anxious, you will become unwell more often than from a casual individual standpoint. Stress can affect your insusceptibility and your risk of diabetes, heart illnesses, and malignant development goes up when you experience continuous pressure. While stress is a side-effect of our cutting-edge way of life, it tends to be defeated with care techniques like pranayama and introspection. Breathing activities help you unwind and deliver pressure that collects throughout some indefinite time range. They likewise support you with interfacing with the parasympathetic sensory system, which is fundamentally an organization of nerves that assist with loosening up your body following occasions of strain or risk. Thus, while mild degrees of stress are crucial for our efficiency, the trouble comes when we can't deliver this pressure efficiently.

How breathing activities assist with managing diabetes

"Stress, uneasiness, and misery are not related to diabetes. 'Endorphins' are delivered when you truly do profound breathing as well as reflection. At the point when you practice pranayama and contemplation routinely, the degrees of counter-administrative chemicals like adrenaline, non-adrenaline, and cortical, which block the activity of insulin decrease. At the point when one does profound breathing, it gets a condition of profound unwinding. The pressure which will in general gather in the muscles, especially in the neck and on one's shoulders, vanishes and one becomes loose and more lively, 10-15 minutes per day of profound breathing will help you in controlling diabetes and furthermore diminishing circulatory strain and forestalling coronary illness,"

Practice proper eating habits and drink a lot of liquids
"L-ascorbic acid and omega unsaturated fats might assist with helping invulnerability. Add jaggery, tulsi, honey, ginger, lemon, basil leaves, and loads of water to your day-to-day diet. Warm water with honey toward the beginning of the day will help,"

Chapter 7: Intermittent Fasting for Improved Insulin Sensitivity and Weight loss.

Intermittent fasting is a form of eating pattern in which you alternate between eating and fasting intervals.

There are many different types of intermittent fasting, such as the 16/8 and 5:2 strategies
Various examinations illustrate the method that can have great advantages for your health and thinking.

The following are 10 proof-based medicinal advantages of intermittent fasting.

1. Changes the capability of substances, cells, and attributes
When you don't eat for a time, a few things happen in your body For instance, your body

changes chemical levels to make the put-away muscle-to-fat ratio more available and initiates substantial cell mending activities.

Here are some of the changes that occur in your body while fasting:

- Insulin levels. Blood levels of insulin decline essentially, which works with fat eating.
- Human development chemical (HGH) levels. Human growth hormone (HGH) levels in the blood may dramatically rise. More heightened levels of this chemical work with fat consumption and muscle gain, and offer numerous varied advantages.
- Cell fix. The body conducts key cell repair activities, such as eliminating waste material from cells Quality articulation. There are favorable alterations in a few characteristics and particles related to life span and disease protection.
- A considerable number of the advantages of discontinuous fasting are associated

with these progressions in chemicals, the capability of cells, and quality articulation.

2. Can assist you with obtaining more fit and more instinctive fat

A considerable majority of folks who undertake discontinuous fasting are doing it to get in shape. Discontinuous fasting, all things considered, will cause you to eat less feasts.

Except if you compensate by eating much more on different nights, you'll end up eating fewer calories.

Moreover, discontinuous fasting increases the chemical capability to operate with weight reduction.

Lower insulin levels, higher HGH levels, and enhanced norepinephrine levels all contribute to the breakdown of muscle vs fat and its usage for energy.

Hence, transitory fasting really expands your metabolic rate, assisting you with ingesting significantly more calories.

All in all, irregular fasting nibbles away at the two sides of the calorie condition. It improves your metabolic rate (burns more calories) and limits the amount of food you eat (diminishes calories in)

As per a 2014 assessment of logical writing, irregular fasting can produce a weight decrease of 3-8% more than 3-24 weeks. This is a tremendous sum.

The review individuals also shed 4-7% of their abdomen circuit more than 6-24 weeks, which suggests that they lost bunches of instinctual fat. Instinctive fat is the painful fat in the stomach hole that causes disease.

One 2011 examination also indicated that irregular fasting generated less muscular deterioration than uninterrupted calorie limitation.

Be that as it may, the 2020 randomized preliminary took a gander at individuals who adopted the 16/8 strategy. In this eating regimen, you quick for 16 hours every day and have an 8-hour window to eat.

folks who refrained didn't shed essentially more weight than folks who ate three dinners every day. In the aftermath of assessing a subgroup of the members face-to-face, the specialists likewise observed that individuals who refrained lost a lot of lean mass. This included fit muscle. More investigations are necessary on the impact of fasting on muscle misfortune. In light of everything, irregular fasting can possibly be an exceptionally strong weight loss apparatus.

3. Can reduce insulin opposition, cutting down your gamble for type 2 diabetes
Type 2 diabetes has transformed into an exceedingly normal conclusion in many years. Its principal comprises excessive glucose levels in relation to insulin opposition.

Whatever minimizes insulin resistance should aid in decreasing glucose levels and protecting against type 2 diabetes.

Curiously, irregular fasting has been exhibited to have considerable advantages for insulin blockage and to trigger an astounding fall in glucose levels (10). In human exams on irregular fasting, fasting glucose has been lowered by 3-6% during the span of 8-12 weeks in individuals with prediabetes. Fasting insulin levels have been lowered by 20-31%.

One concentrate in mice with diabetes moreover demonstrated that discontinuous fasting further grew endurance rates and protected against diabetic retinopathy. Diabetic retinopathy is a discomfort that might trigger a visual deficit.

What this infers is that discontinuous fasting might be extremely defensive for individuals who are in danger of getting type 2 diabetes.
Be that as it may, there might be a few distinctions between the genders. One 2005

concentration on ladies indicated that glucose in the executives actually disintegrated following a 22-day-long irregular fasting convention.

4. Can lessen oxidative pressure and aggravation in the body

Oxidative pressure is one of the strategies for developing various continuous ailments.

It comprises unsteady atoms dubbed free extremists. Free revolutionaries respond with other critical atoms, like protein and DNA, and harm them. A few examinations demonstrate that irregular fasting might increase the body's resistance to oxidative pressure.

Moreover, concentrates on demonstrating the way that discontinuous fasting might assist with battling irritation, one more major driver of numerous regular infections.

5. Might be useful for heart wellness

Coronary sickness is right now the world's greatest executioner.

It's acknowledged that diverse well-being markers (purported "risk factors") are associated with either an extended or lessened likelihood of cardiovascular sickness.

Discontinuous fasting has been exhibited to further develop numerous different gambling elements, including:

- glucose levels
- circulatory strain
- blood fatty substances
- aggregate and LDL (bad) cholesterol
- flaming markers

Notwithstanding, a lot of this relies on creature studies.

The effects of fasting on heart well-being should be concentrated from top to bottom in people before suggestions can be made.

6. Instigates various cell fix processes

At the moment where we quick, the phones in the body start a phone "squander expulsion" activity called autophagy

This comprises the cells sorting and utilizing damaged and useless proteins that grow inside cells after some period.

Expanded autophagy may give security against a few infections, including malignant development and neurological illnesses like Alzheimer's illness.

7. May assist with forestalling sickness

The condition is characterized by the unregulated development of cells.

Fasting has been exhibited to affect digestion which would prompt lessened hazard of sickness.

Promising data from creature studies suggests that discontinuous fasting or diets that duplicate fasting might assist with forestalling sickness.

Research in humans has led to comparative discoveries, however, additional exams are required.

There's also some proof that fasting lessened different symptoms of chemotherapy in folks.

8. Has benefits for your cerebrum

What's terrific for the body is a lot of the time great for the cerebrum also.

Irregular fasting further develops numerous metabolic elements considered to be vital for cerebrum well-being.

Irregular fasting diminishes:

- oxidative pressure
- irritation
- glucose levels
- insulin opposition

A few examinations in mice and rodents have revealed that irregular fasting might enhance the formation of new nerve cells, which ought to have benefits for cerebrum capability.

Fasting likewise develops levels of a cerebrum substance called mind-inferred neurotrophic factor
(BDNF). A shortage of BDNF has been involved in gloom and numerous other cerebrum disorders.

Creature investigations have likewise indicated that irregular fasting shields against mental harm because of strokes

9. May aid with forestalling Alzheimer's infection

Alzheimer's sickness is the world's most normal neurodegenerative infection.

There's no repair at present accessible for Alzheimer's, so stopping it from showing, in any case, is basic.

Concentrations on rodents and mice reveal that discontinuous fasting might postpone the beginning of Alzheimer's or diminish its seriousness.

In a progression of case reports, a way of life mediation that incorporated everyday momentary diets had the ability to essentially work on Alzheimer's side effects in 9 out of 10 individuals.

Creature concentrations additionally propose that fasting might shield against different neurodegenerative infections, including Parkinson's sickness and Huntington's sicknesses.

10. May extend your life expectancy, supporting you with living longer

One of the most fascinating utilizations of discontinuous fasting would be its capacity to widen life expectancy.

Concentrates on rodents have indicated that discontinuous fasting enhances life expectancy along these lines as continual calorie limitation

Discontinuous fasting has likewise been exhibited to raise the life expectancies of organic product flies.

In a piece of these exams, the impacts were quite sensational. In a more seasoned study, rats who refrained each and every other day lived 83% longer than rodents who didn't abstain (44).

In a recent investigation, mice that abstained each and every other day had their life expectancies increase by roughly 13%.

Day-to-day fasting was also exhibited to work on the general well-being of male mice. It helped postpone the onset of illnesses like greasy liver disease and hepatocellular carcinoma, which are both normal in aging mic

Albeit this is a long way not fully resolved in individuals, discontinuous fasting has been exceptionally famous amid the counter-maturing swarm.

Given the established advantages for digestion and a wide range of well-being markers, it's a solid concept that irregular fasting could assist you with keeping on with a more drawn-out and happier existence.

Discontinuous Fasting for Genuine Individuals: Functional Tips to Eat on Time

Irregular fasting (IF) has been around for some time. It took a significant rise in fame back in 2013 with "The 8-Hour Diet" by David Zinczenko and Peter Moore.

Before sufficiently long, superstars like Hugh Jackman, Beyoncé, Nicole Kidman, Miranda Kerr, and Benedict Cumberbatch were all supposedly taken on some sort of the IF diet.

The eating regimen entails limiting the time span in which you eat food. As a way, you go through rotating periods of fasting and eating. Dissimilar to most distinct weight control strategies, it's connected with regulating when you eat as opposed to what you eat.

Different exams have revealed that by taking on this eating design, you could experience benefits like:

- weight decrease
- worked on metabolic wellbeing
- security from disease
- a greater longer life range

On the off chance that you're eager to attempt this moving eating plan, you could be a little stressed about exactly the way in which you'll oversee it.

It's one thing to go into a restrictive eating program as a celebrity with an own dietician. It's considerably harder when you have things like your work or your children to shuffle simultaneously!

Peruse on to locate a few effective suggestions and deceives that everyone may use to begin consuming an IF regimen.

Getting everything rolling. You realize you need to attempt IF, however, perhaps you don't know where to begin.

Priorities straight: Properly investigate topics. As nutritionist, Stephanie Rofkahr from Fit Four Five makes sense of, On the off chance that it is harmful to individuals with low glucose. Converse with your main care physician before you roll out any adjustments to your eating regimen.

Then, conclude which kind to attempt. There are six well-known fasting examples to go over, although this rundown is in no way, shape, or form exhaustive.

Whenever you've examined as needed and settled on the timetable that turns out best for you, you're all set.

Ways to keep it managed
Assuming that can be severe, particularly to start with. Notwithstanding the evident protesting of

your stomach, you may likewise confront fatigue, peevishness, and worry when you attempt to deal with your new eating plan.

Here are a few ideas to make your life considerably simpler:

* **Begin with a revised timetable**. "Begin with a timetable that is reasonable for yourself and

thereafter add onto the power and term, "set out nutritionists at Nucific. Don't bother making a plunge! Fabricate your resistance to eating in a more modest time window every day, then tackle the entire timetable when you're prepared.

* **Remain all-around hydrated**. Lee makes sense that you ought to continue hydrating with "noncaloric liquids" during your fasting phase. This can involve water, natural teas, and sans-calorie seasoned drinks.

* **During the eating time frame, eat gently and often.** Rofkahr advises that you aim to eat

like clockwork inside the 8-hour window so you can "get your calories in." Recollect that IF might become dangerous in the event that you don't acquire your indicated everyday calorie consumption.

* **Plan sound, nutritious feasts early.** While you might be attracted to indulge yourself with your number one snack and consolation food sources when your fasting period is done, endeavor to adhere to a solid eating routine with proteins, natural goods, and vegetables.

* **Prepare your feasts ahead of time**. In the event that your timetable is excessively packed, put away the opportunity near the end of the week or a couple of evenings seven days to set up key feasts ahead of time. This will save you time and assist you with keeping your eating regimen regulated.

* **Add 2 to 3 tbsp**. of solid fat to your night dinner. Alicia Galvin, RD, an accredited dietician for Sovereign Research centers,

advocates eating a healthy fat like olive oil, coconut spread, or avocado in the last dinner of the day to keep glucose levels steady short-term.

*** Assuming you experience difficulties napping** IF probably won't be for you. As suggested by IF instructor Cynthia Thurlow, "On the off chance that you can't stay asleep from sundown to sunset, don't endeavor to utilize this methodology. Work on rest first."

Chapter 8: Exercise and Insulin Sensitivity

Regardless of the form of diabetes — pre-diabetes, gestational diabetes, type 1 diabetes, or type 2 diabetes — practice is usually suggested to support wonderful well-being. While practice is associated with further increasing cardiovascular hazard factors, weight reduction initiatives, and physical and mental prosperity, it is exercise's effect on blood glucose control that routinely rouses many would-be sedentary people with diabetes to get up and move.

Insulin awareness is your body's ability to haul glucose out of the circulatory system and place it into your cells with the goal that glucose can be utilized for energy or fuel for the cell. While glucose is absolutely not something horrible, a lot of glucose is certainly not something to be pleased with. Controlling blood glucose is associated with solid results.

Remembering exercise for your everyday plan can lessen blood glucose and return to maintaining glucose within a sound target reach. While you might feel overpowered and would prefer to search down a cause than a rec center, no genuine reasons. Simply move!
Practice boosts insulin awareness during the genuine actual work as well as soon after that action called practice recuperation. Practice recuperation could be a matter of moments or a few hours lengthy.

The impact of the activity on insulin awareness could fluctuate from the accompanying:

* **Recurrence of actual work:** Exercise-incited insulin response declines after the action. This reality alone backs practicing consistently.

* **Force and span of actual labor:** Power, how testing the action is to the individual, and

duration, the time working out, might be the best powerhouse of insulin response during and post work out. A long-length action performed at a low or simple power can be filled in for a brief-term movement performed at a greater or seriously stimulating power to accomplish comparative metabolic consequences and insulin responsiveness findings. An illustration of this may be the movement of working in the nursery for two to four hours contrasted with a thirty to hour-long walk. While length and power are radically different, the results could be almost the same. No actual reasons. Move!
Kind of actual work: many choices are dynamic:

* **High-impact practice upholds expanded perseverance and incorporates ongoing growth of big muscle groupings.** High-impact action increases your pulse and makes you breathe more quickly.

* **Loads/obstruction procedures generate muscular contraction against an outside force.** The outside power could be as

straightforward as lifting one's arms as well as legs, leg squats, or potentially moving back and forth against a weight or blockage group.

*** Adaptability and Equilibrium work out, while sluggish and pondering, support a wide scope of mobility and harm prevention.**

There is outstanding individual changeability to the actual job and insulin responsiveness. By composing notes in your logbook, you will start to see designs arise. A certain form of action may not affect blood glucose. Another activity will in general drop glucose for quite a long time. The most effective strategy to organize your reaction to practice is to save basic notes and hunt for rehashed designs. You will likewise realize that glucose observing will have more significant worth as you can examine the distinction diverse exercises have on your blood glucose. Take the logbook with you to the specialist and present your disclosures. There's positively no size fits generally here. Moreover, the support of a credentialed diabetic care and training specialist is profitable while learning the importance of the examples you experience.

In the event that you end up sitting before a PC screen the majority of the day, committed time for the actual job may not appear to be doable. Keep in mind: no good justifications. Everybody can follow through with something. Have a go at standing up and extending each ten to fifteen minutes (add a suggestion to your phone or set a caution); when you walk anyplace, walk tall with shoulders pulled somewhat back; don't take the lift for a solitary floor, use the stairwell; rather than strolling to the nearest bathroom, go to a more far off area; and whenever you leave the car, leave away from the entry and get somewhat more movement while traveling every which way. Primary concern: in the event that you can't zero in on being more active then, at that point, revolve around being less dormant. That is to say, whenever you get an opportunity to move and stretch your body during your day then, at that point, move. To put it bluntly, it's all actual development, that improves well-being and insulin awareness.

Make sure to exercise on many instances a day routinely regardless of whether merely for a couple of moments each time (easily missed subtleties really do add up!). Development is exercise and as you work out, your body builds its capacity to transport glucose into your cells and utilize that glucose for energy. This interest in insulin awareness brings down glucose when you're practicing as well as interest into the period thereafter. Assuming you're training consistently, insulin demands will decline and you'll find it simpler to keep blood sugars within your aim reach.

No actual reasons. Focus on keeping away from significant stretches of idleness regularly. You'll feel quite a little improved at the day's end!

Chapter 8: Physical Activity and Diabetes

Physical activity is a game-changer when it comes to managing diabetes. It's not just about breaking a sweat; it's a powerful tool that can positively impact your blood sugar levels and overall well-being. In this chapter, we'll explore the incredible benefits of exercise for diabetes management and discover the types of activities that work best for different types of diabetes, how you can create ur personal exercise plan, and how to overcome its challenges.

Benefits of Exercise for Diabetes Management

Exercise is like a superhero for your body, especially when it comes to diabetes. Here are some of the remarkable benefits:

* **Improved Insulin Sensitivity**: When you engage in regular physical activity, your cells become more responsive to insulin. This means your body can use insulin more effectively to lower blood sugar levels.

* **Blood Sugar Regulation:** Exercise helps regulate blood sugar levels by promoting the uptake of glucose by your muscles. This not only reduces immediate spikes but also contributes to better long-term control.

* **Weight Management**: When it comes to managing diabetes, maintaining a healthy weight is so crucial and essential. Exercise helps burn calories, making it a key player in weight management and reducing the risk of obesity-related complications.

* **Heart Health**: Diabetes and heart issues often go hand in hand. Regular exercise strengthens the heart, improves circulation, and lowers the risk of cardiovascular diseases, a significant concern for individuals with diabetes.

* **Stress Reduction:** Stress can wreak havoc on blood sugar levels. Exercise acts as a natural stress reliever, releasing endorphins that improve mood and reduce stress, ultimately benefiting diabetes management.

* **Improved Sleep:** Quality sleep is vital for overall health and diabetes management. Exercise contributes to better sleep patterns, creating a positive cycle of improved energy levels and glucose regulation.

* **Muscle Health:** Building and maintaining muscle through exercise enhances overall metabolism. This can be a benefit for individuals with Type 2 diabetes or Insulin resistance.

* **Enhanced Blood Circulation**: Good circulation is essential for delivering nutrients and oxygen throughout the body. Exercise improves blood flow, supporting the health of various organs and tissues.

Types of Exercise Suitable for Different Types of Diabetes

Exercise is not one-size-fits-all, and the same goes for diabetes. Tailoring your physical activity to your specific type of diabetes is key. Here's a breakdown:

Type 1 Diabetes:

- **Aerobic Exercise**: Activities like walking, jogging, or cycling are excellent for cardiovascular health.
- **Strength Training**: Incorporating resistance exercises helps build muscle and can enhance insulin sensitivity.

Type 1.5 Diabetes:

- **Combination Exercises**: Opt for workouts that combine both aerobic and strength training elements to address the characteristics of both Type 1 and Type 2 diabetes.

Type 2 Diabetes:

- **Moderate Aerobic Exercise:** Brisk walking, swimming, or dancing can help improve insulin sensitivity without putting excessive strain on the body.
- **Resistance Training:** Building muscle mass aids in glucose uptake, making resistance training beneficial.

Prediabetes:

- **Gradual Progression:** Start with low-impact activities like walking and gradually incorporate more intense exercises as fitness improves.
- **Consistency is Key:** Regular, moderate exercise is crucial for preventing the progression of Type 2 diabetes.

Gestational Diabetes:

- **Prenatal Exercises:** Safe, low-impact activities like prenatal yoga or swimming can help manage blood sugar levels during pregnancy.
- **Consultation with Healthcare Providers**: Always consult with healthcare providers to ensure exercise plans align with the specific needs of pregnancy and gestational diabetes.

Remember, the key is finding activities you enjoy and can sustain over time. Whether it's dancing, hiking, or gardening, the goal is to keep moving. So, lace up those sneakers, find your rhythm, and let the benefits of physical activity work their magic in your diabetes management journey.

Creating an Individualized Exercise Plan

When it comes to managing diabetes, incorporating physical activity is like giving your body a superhero boost. Exercise not only helps control blood sugar levels but also enhances insulin sensitivity. The key is to craft an exercise plan tailored to your unique needs and preferences.

Start by considering your fitness level and any existing health conditions. If you're new to exercise or have physical limitations, begin with low-impact activities such as walking, swimming, or cycling. These gentle forms of exercise lay a solid foundation for more intense workouts down the road.

For those already familiar with regular exercise, the focus shifts to variety and intensity. A well-rounded routine includes both aerobic exercises, like jogging or dancing, and strength training, such as weightlifting or yoga. Aerobic exercises elevate your heart rate, burning calories and improving cardiovascular health. Strength training, on the other hand, builds muscle, boosting your body's ability to manage glucose.

Consistency is key. Aim for two times a week at least in strength training exercises in addition to 150 minutes or more of moderate-intensity aerobic activity per week. However, always listen to your body. If you're feeling fatigued or unwell, it's okay to take a break and resume when you're ready.

Remember, there's no one-size-fits-all solution. Your exercise plan should align with your lifestyle and preferences. If you enjoy the great outdoors, consider activities like hiking or biking. If you prefer the comfort of your home, explore online workout classes or invest in home gym equipment.

Lastly, involve a mix of activities to keep things interesting. This keeps you from becoming bored and guarantees that you are using diverse muscle groups. From dancing to gardening, find what brings you joy, and let that be the driving force behind your exercise routine.

Overcoming Barriers to Physical Activity

Embarking on an exercise journey can be daunting, especially when faced with obstacles that threaten to derail your efforts. Let's tackle some common barriers and pave the way for a more active lifestyle.

1. Time Constraints: In the hustle and bustle of daily life, finding time for exercise can seem impossible. The solution? Schedule it like any other appointment. Whether it's a morning walk or an evening workout, mark it on your calendar. Treat it with the same importance as a work meeting or a family gathering.

2. Lack of Motivation: Staying motivated is a universal challenge. Combat this by setting realistic goals. Start small, celebrate achievements, and gradually increase the intensity. Consider finding a workout buddy for mutual encouragement, or make your favorite music the backdrop to your exercise routine.

3. Physical Limitations: Chronic conditions or physical restrictions may make certain activities challenging. The key is to find exercises that accommodate your abilities. Chair exercises, water aerobics, or seated yoga are excellent options for those with mobility issues. Always consult with your healthcare provider to ensure your chosen activities are safe and beneficial.

4. Weather Concerns: Unpredictable weather can be a deterrent, especially for outdoor activities. Have a backup plan for indoor exercises, whether it's a home workout routine or a gym session. This way, you're not at the mercy of the weather, ensuring consistency in your fitness routine.

5. Fear of Injury: The fear of getting hurt can be paralyzing. Start slowly and prioritize proper form over intensity. If you're unsure about specific exercises, seek guidance from a fitness professional. Gradually build up your strength and confidence, and don't be afraid to modify exercises to suit your comfort level.

6. Financial Constraints: You don't need a fancy gym membership or expensive equipment to stay active. Many efficient exercises require little or no equipment. Walking, jogging, bodyweight exercises, and online workout videos are budget-friendly alternatives. Get creative with what you have, and remember, the most important investment is your commitment to moving your body.

By acknowledging and addressing these barriers, you pave the way for a sustainable and enjoyable exercise routine. Remember, the journey to mastering diabetes is a marathon, not a sprint. With the right mindset and a personalized plan, you're not just managing diabetes—you're thriving.

Chapter 9: Nutritional Strategies for Diabetes Control

Low-carb vs. Balanced Diets

Many people navigating the realm of diabetes management often find themselves at a crossroads when it comes to choosing the right diet. The age-old debate between low-carb and balanced diets takes center stage. Let's demystify the choices.

Low-Carb Diets:

Imagine your body as a high-performance car. Low-carb diets are like providing it with the premium fuel it needs to function optimally. In the context of diabetes, restricting carbohydrates helps manage blood sugar levels more effectively. By minimizing the intake of sugars and refined carbs, you're essentially removing the fast-burning twigs from your metabolic fire. This prevents sudden spikes in blood sugar, making it easier for your body to process and utilize insulin.

But remember, not all carbs are created equal. While slashing the intake of processed carbs is crucial, whole grains, vegetables, and fruits should still find a place on your plate. They bring along a wealth of essential nutrients, fiber, and slow-releasing energy, ensuring your body runs smoothly over the long haul.

Balanced Diets:

Now, think of a balanced diet as the conductor orchestrating a symphony within your body. It's all about variety, moderation, and harmony. A balanced diet doesn't vilify any particular macronutrient but rather emphasizes a mix of carbohydrates, proteins, and fats. This approach ensures a steady and sustained release of energy, helping to keep blood sugar levels stable.

For individuals with diabetes, a balanced diet offers flexibility and a broader spectrum of nutrients. It's like giving your body a well-rounded toolkit to deal with the intricacies of metabolism. The key is in portion control and choosing the right sources for each macronutrient. Whole grains, lean proteins, and healthy fats become your allies in maintaining a delicate balance between nourishment and blood sugar control.

In the end, the choice between low-carb and balanced diets boils down to personal preferences, metabolic responses, and lifestyle. It's not about adopting a one-size-fits-all approach but rather understanding what resonates best with your body's unique needs.

The Role of Fiber, Protein, and Healthy Fats

Now that we've dipped our toes into the dietary debate, let's dive deeper into the triumvirate of nutrition—fiber, protein, and healthy fats. These elements are the unsung heroes in the battle against diabetes.

Fiber:

Picture fiber as the broom sweeping away excess sugar and cholesterol from your body. Found abundantly in fruits, vegetables, whole grains, and legumes, fiber is a powerhouse of health benefits. For individuals managing diabetes, fiber acts as a natural blood sugar regulator. It slows down the digestion and absorption of sugars, preventing abrupt spikes.

Moreover, fiber is your gut's best friend. A healthy gut contributes to improved insulin sensitivity, creating a positive ripple effect on your overall metabolic well-being. So, don't shy away from those colorful salads, whole grains, and crunchy vegetables—your body will thank you for the fiber boost.

Protein:

Proteins are the building blocks of life, and in the context of diabetes, they play a crucial role in stabilizing blood sugar levels. When you consume protein-rich foods like lean meats, fish, eggs, dairy, legumes, and nuts, you provide your body with a sustained source of energy.

Proteins also aid in muscle development and repair, contributing to a healthier body composition. This is particularly important for individuals with diabetes, as maintaining muscle mass can enhance insulin sensitivity. So, think of protein as the reliable friend who's got your back, helping you navigate the ups and downs of blood sugar management.

Healthy Fats:

Contrary to the outdated notion that all fats are foes, the right kinds of fats can be your allies in the fight against diabetes. Healthy fats, found in avocados, nuts, seeds, olive oil, and fatty fish, boast an impressive resume of benefits.

These fats play a pivotal role in satiety, keeping you full and satisfied for longer periods. This can be a game-changer in preventing overeating and managing weight—an essential aspect of diabetes control. Additionally, healthy fats contribute to improved heart health, an often-overlooked aspect for those with diabetes who may be at a higher risk of cardiovascular issues.

In essence, think of fiber, protein, and healthy fats as the dynamic trio ensuring your body's metabolic orchestra performs a harmonious symphony. They not only contribute to blood sugar regulation but also bring a plethora of additional health benefits to the diabetes management table. So, embrace the rainbow of whole foods and let your plate become a canvas of nutritional artistry.

Glycemic Index and Its Implications

Understanding the Glycemic Index (GI) is like having a secret decoder for managing diabetes through food. It's not about avoiding all carbs, but rather choosing the right ones to keep your blood sugar levels steady. Let's break it down in simpler terms.

Imagine your body as a finely tuned engine, and the food you eat as the fuel. The Glycemic Index is a ranking system that tells you how quickly certain foods raise your blood sugar. Foods with a high GI are like rocket fuel, causing a rapid spike, while low-GI foods are like slow-burning logs that provide a steady release of energy.

In the world of diabetes mastery, the goal is to focus on low-GI foods to prevent sudden spikes in blood sugar levels. These foods are your allies in the battle against insulin resistance. Opting for whole grains, legumes, non-starchy vegetables, and fruits with a lower GI can help keep your blood sugar levels on an even keel.

Take oatmeal, for instance. A bowl of steel-cut oats has a lower GI than instant oatmeal packets. Why does this matter? Because the slower release of energy from the steel-cut oats means a gentler impact on your blood sugar levels. It's not about avoiding oatmeal altogether but making a savvy choice that aligns with your body's needs.

But wait, there's more to the story than just numbers. Pairing high-GI foods with low-GI foods can also be a smart strategy. For example, adding healthy fats or protein to your meal can slow down the absorption of carbohydrates, mitigating the overall impact on blood sugar levels. It's like assembling a team of foods that work together to keep your metabolism in check.

So, the next time you're at the grocery store or planning your meals, think beyond counting carbs. Consider the glycemic impact of what you're about to eat, and you'll be one step closer to mastering diabetes through smart nutritional choices.

Meal Planning for Diabetes Mastery

Meal planning doesn't have to be a daunting task; in fact, it can be your secret weapon in the fight against diabetes. Picture it as a roadmap for your day, guiding you to make food choices that support your health goals. Let's unravel the art of meal planning in the context of diabetes mastery.

1. Variety is Your Spice of Life:
One of the keys to successful meal planning is embracing a diverse range of foods. Don't limit yourself to a monotonous routine. Mix it up with a rainbow of vegetables, lean proteins, whole grains, and healthy fats. Variety not only makes your meals more enjoyable but also ensures you get a broad spectrum of nutrients.

2. Portion Control Matters:
It's not just what you eat but how much that counts. Portion control is your ally in managing blood sugar levels. Rather than piling your plate high, savor smaller portions that balance

carbohydrates, proteins, and fats. This not only helps regulate blood sugar but also prevents overeating, supporting overall health.

3. Timing is Everything:

Eating at consistent times each day can help stabilize blood sugar levels. Aim for three balanced meals and include healthy snacks if needed. This steady rhythm helps your body anticipate and manage the incoming fuel, preventing sudden spikes or crashes. Consistency is the name of the game.

4. The Power of Pre-Planning:

Has the adage "Failing to plan is planning to fail" ever occurred to you? It holds true for meal planning too. Take some time each week to outline your meals, create a shopping list, and prepare what you can in advance. Having healthy options readily available makes it easier to resist the temptation of less desirable choices.

5. Embrace the Plate Method:

A simple yet effective approach to meal planning is the plate method. Visualize your plate divided into sections: half for non-starchy vegetables, a quarter for lean protein, and a quarter for whole grains or starchy vegetables. This method not only simplifies portioning but also ensures a well-balanced and diabetes-friendly meal.

6. Hydrate Wisely:
Don't forget about hydration in your meal planning strategy. Opt for water or other low-calorie beverages over sugary drinks. Proper hydration supports overall health and can even help regulate appetite, making it a crucial component of your mealtime routine.

In the world of diabetes mastery, meal planning is your ally, not a restrictive rulebook. It's about making thoughtful choices that align with your body's needs and your health goals. So, let your creativity shine in the kitchen, experiment with flavors, and savor the journey of mastering diabetes one delicious and well-planned meal at a time.

Overseeing glucose levels is crucial to living fantastic with diabetes and staying away from a piece of its complications. Keeping a sound food regimen can help. Following a diabetes feast plan can aid an individual with assuring assortment in their eating regimen and help them in coming to or holding a moderate weight.
This post presents two 7-day meal menus appropriate for those on a calorie-controlled distrusted Source to promote weight reduction. One delivers 1,200 calories each day and the other gives 1,600 every day.

Be that as it may, nobody's strategy will suit everybody. At last, it is advisable for every individual to set out their own supper plan with support from a professional or dietician.
Bit-by-bit instructions

Individuals with diabetes might join in a healthy, changed diet that assists with regulating glucose levels.

Fostering this kind of diet includes:

- modifying carbohydrates, proteins, and lipids to achieve nutritional objectives
- estimating portions precisely
- Preparing

In view of this, the accompanying advancements might assist a person with assembling a good 7-day dinner plan:

- Note every day focuses on calories and carbs.
- Decide the number of parts of carbs and other meal components that will achieve those aims.
- Split those components throughout a day's feasts and snacks.
- Survey the ranks of #1 and identifiable food kinds and strive to combine them

into dinners, taking into account the data above.

- Trade records bunch food sources as per the number of carbohydrates they contain, simplifying it to trade one food type for another. They may likewise cluster food sources with comparable degrees of fats and proteins and integrate subcategories.
- Plan feasts to magnify fixing use, for example, by having cook chicken one day and chicken soup the following.
- Rehash the interaction for every day of the week.
- Screen glucose levels every day and weight consistently to examine whether the arrangement is producing the optimal outcomes.

Factors impacting dietary decisions for patients with diabetes include:

- balancing starch consumption with activity levels and the utilization of insulin and various medicines

- ingesting a lot of fiber to assist in managing trustworthy Sources with blooding sugar levels
- limiting profoundly handled starches and dietary sources with added sugars
- knowing what dietary decisions can signify for entanglements of diabetes, for example, hypertension
- managing weight by considering individual treatment programs and ideas from a specialist or nutritionist
- Consolidating the different approaches beneath may help generate a diabetes dinner plan.

Weight management

They have all the earmarks of being a linkTrusted Source among diabetes and heftiness. Many persons with diabetes can be meaning to acquire more fit or forestall weight increase.

One approach for controlling weight can be by calculating calories. The quantity of calories an individual requires every day will rely upon aspects, for example,

- blood glucose goals
- action levels
- level
- sex
- specific designs to reduce, acquire, or keep up with weight
- the utilization of insulin and alternative medications
- inclinations
- expenditure plan

Different dietary approaches might assist an individual in reaching and sustaining a moderate weight, and not every one of them contains calculating calories.

The Scramble diet, for instance, revolves largely around organic food, vegetables, entire grains, nuts, and seeds, as well as dairy items, poultry, and fish that are low in fat or sans fat. It instructs individuals to steer away from additional salt, sweets, undesirable fats, red meat and handled carbs.

The Scramble diet indicates further expanded pulse levels in individuals with hypertension, although research Source additionally recommends it might aid with shedding and controlling weight.

Be that as it may, nobody's strategy will suit everybody. At last, it is advisable for every individual to resolve their own supper plan with guidance from a specialist or dietician.

7 Days Diabetes Meal plan

The foods you eat play a crucial role in managing blood sugar levels and improving insulin sensitivity. Let's dive into a practical and delicious 7-day diabetes meal plan to help you take charge of your health.

Day 1: Balanced Beginnings

- **Breakfast**: Kickstart your day with a bowl of oatmeal topped with fresh berries and a sprinkle of chia seeds. .

- **Lunch**: Opt for a colorful salad with leafy greens, cherry tomatoes, cucumbers, and grilled chicken. Dress it with olive oil and balsamic vinegar.

- **Dinner**: Enjoy a serving of grilled salmon with steamed broccoli and quinoa. This nutrient-rich dinner will keep you satisfied without causing blood sugar spikes.

Day 2: Veggie Power

- **Breakfast**: Try a vegetable omelet with spinach, bell peppers, and tomatoes. Serve it with a slice of whole-grain toast.Eat it with a boiled egg to increase your protein intake.

- **Lunch**: Have a hearty bowl of lentil soup and a side of mixed greens. Lentils provide a good source of protein and fiber.

- **Dinner**: Roast a variety of colorful vegetables such as carrots, sweet potatoes, and Brussels sprouts. Add a grilled chicken breast for a well-rounded meal.

Day 3: Mediterranean Flavors

- **Breakfast**: Greek yogurt with sliced peaches and a drizzle of honey makes for a delightful and protein-packed breakfast.

- **Lunch**: Prepare a Mediterranean-inspired salad with feta cheese, olives, cherry tomatoes, and grilled shrimp.

- **Dinner**: Indulge in a piece of grilled white fish (like cod or tilapia) with a side of quinoa and roasted asparagus.

Day 4: Plant-Powered Delights

- **Breakfast**: Blend a green smoothie with kale, banana, and almond milk for a nutrient-packed start to your day.

- **Lunch**: Enjoy a chickpea and vegetable stir-fry with a light soy sauce. Serve it over brown rice or cauliflower rice.

- **Dinner**: Roasted vegetable and black bean enchiladas with a side of guacamole make for a flavorful and satisfying dinner.

Day 5: Lean and Green

- **Breakfast**: Scramble some eggs with spinach and mushrooms. Pair it with a slice of whole-grain toast.

- **Lunch**: Opt for a grilled chicken salad with mixed greens, cherry tomatoes, and a tangy vinaigrette dressing.

- **Dinner**: Grill a lean steak and serve it with a side of roasted Brussels sprouts and quinoa.

Day 6: Comforting Classics

- **Breakfast**: Whole-grain pancakes topped with sliced bananas and a dollop of Greek yogurt are a delicious way to start your day.

- **Lunch**: Make a whole-grain tortilla wrap with turkey and avocado. Add plenty of fresh veggies for extra crunch.

- **Dinner**: Bake a piece of salmon with lemon and herbs, and pair it with sweet potato wedges and steamed green beans.

Day 7: Wholesome Indulgence

- **Breakfast**: Enjoy a parfait made with layers of Greek yogurt, granola, and mixed berries.

- **Lunch**: Treat yourself to a quinoa and black bean bowl with avocado and salsa.

- **Dinner**: Savor a comforting bowl of vegetable and lentil stew. Add a side of whole-grain bread for a complete meal.

Creating a variety of delicious and nutritious meals is the key to sustainable diabetes management. Experiment with flavors, discover what works best for your taste buds, and embrace the journey to mastering diabetes through mindful and enjoyable eating.

Chapter 10: Delicious and Healthful Dishes for Reducing Blood Bugar Levels

A diabetes diet can be made sound as well as enjoyable with solid fixes. The following are 6 delectable diabetes-accommodating recipes you should attempt at home.

Living with diabetes doesn't imply one can't appreciate taste alongside well-being. All you require is a shift to sound and low GI fixes.

Individuals with diabetes usually complain about the absence of flavor and taste in their meals as they need to follow a severe solid eating routine absent any trace of sugar, carbohydrates, and soaking fats that they delighted in indiscriminately before they were determined to have the sickness. Nonetheless, living with diabetes doesn't imply one can't appreciate taste with well-being. All you want is a shift to solid and low GI fixes with high protein, fiber, and heaps of cell reinforcements to hold your sugar levels under wraps. Changing to entire grains, solid spices, and flavors, low-fat dairy, and green and verdant vegetables will as a matter of fact change up

your plate and you can fall head over heels for your diabetes diet more than your customary eating regimen in the event that you plan your dinners ahead of time.

The following are 6 diabetes-accommodating solid recipes:

1. Fiery coconut shrimp (Asian)
Ingredients:

1 cup quinoa, flushed. 2 glasses of water. 1/4 teaspoon salt

shrimp:
1 teaspoon olive oil. 1 medium onion, slashed. 1 tablespoon minced new ginger root. 1/2

teaspoon curry powder. 1/2 teaspoon ground cumin. 1/4 teaspoon salt. 1/4 teaspoon cayenne pepper.

1 pound uncooked shrimp (26-30 per pound), deveined and stripped .. 2 cups young snow peas (about 7 ounces), handled.. 3 tablespoons light coconut milk

1 tablespoon squeezed orange. 1/4 cup improved destroyed coconut, toasted.. 1/4 cup minced new cilantro

Method

- In a big pan, join quinoa, water, and salt; heat to the point of boiling.
- Decrease heat; stew, covered, 12-15 minutes or until fluid is retained.
- Eliminate heat; cushion with a fork.
- In the meantime, in an enormous nonstick skillet, heat oil over medium intensity. Add onion; heat and stir for 4-6 minutes or until delicate. Mix in ginger, curry powder, cumin, salt, and cayenne; heat for a little period.
- Add shrimp and snow peas to skillet; heat and combine

about 3-4 minutes or until shrimp become pink and snow peas are fresh and delicate.

- Mix in coconut milk and squeezed orange; heat through. Present with quinoa; top each presenting with coconut and cilantro.

2. Goan Prawn Curry (Goan Sambharachi Kodi) (Indian)

Ingredients:

1 kilogram of cleaned and shelled prawns. Drudgery to glue.. 1 ground coconut.. 4 dry red chilies.. 1-loaded tsp cumin.. ½ tsp turmeric powder Pound together

3-4 chilies. ¾ tamarind water (prepared with a lime-sized ½ inch slice of a ginger wad of tamarind). 1 larger slashed onion. Salt to taste

Method

- Blend the masala glue and the squashed masala together in a dish and simmer, adding water at whatever point is necessary, for around 20 minutes.

- Then, at that point, add the cleaned and shelled prawns to which salt has been added and stew till the prawns are done.

3. Dahi wali bhindi (Indian)

Ingredients:
4 tbsp vegetable oil.. 1 cup onion cubed.. 400 g bhindi.. 1 tsp cumin seeds.. ¼ tsp Hing.. 2 tsp ginger garlic glue.. 2-3 green chilies sliced into half. 1 tsp coriander powder.. ½ tsp turmeric powder.. 2 tsp Kashmiri red bean stew powder.. ½ tsp cumin powder. Salt to taste.. 1 cup yogurt.. 1 tsp normal baking flour.. ½ tsp garam masala powder

Method
- Using a kitchen towel, wash and dry the bhindi.
- Cut them into 1-inch length pieces.
- Heat oil in a container.
- Add bhindi and sear till they are fairly caramelized.
- Channel on a platter.

- Add onion and fry till they are perfectly done.
- Add cumin seeds and hing and sear for a couple of seconds
- Presently add ginger-garlic glue and green stew and heat for 2-3 minutes.
- Add ½ cup water and boil quickly.
- Add coriander powder, turmeric powder, red stew powder, cumin powder, and salt to taste and simmer quickly.
- Whisk yogurt with ordinary baking flour add it to the dish and cook for 2-3 minutes until the oil begins to isolate from the sides.
- Add broiled bhindi and 1 cup of water and simmer for 3-4 minutes.
- Stir in the garam masala powder
- Decorate with new coriander and serve hot.

Take Note:
Continuously appropriately wash okra and dry it with a kitchen towel. Rest it for somewhere around 30 minutes prior to applying it to forestall sludge in Bhindi.
Utilize well-whisked yogurt for putting up the curry. Try not to add the yogurt in its regular

structure as it probably won't produce a smooth and velvety top to the sauce.

Likewise, toss charred okra into the curry without a second to spare or only a handful of moments before at long last serving it.

4. Chargrilled fish with green stew, coriander, and coconut relish (Western)

Ingredients:

1 tiny red onion, thinly slashed.. 1 tsp finely ground new ginger.. 1 tsp mustard seeds.. 20g (1/4 cup) destroyed coconut.. 1 bracket tomato, cultivated, carefully slashed.. 1 long young green bean stew, farmed, meagerly sliced.. 1/4 cup hacked new coriander.. 1 tbsp lime juice. Touch of caster sugar.. 4 (about 150g each) firm white fish filets. To serve: steamed green beans. Steam-roasted asparagus, ready to eat

Methods:

- Heat a griddle over medium intensity. Shower with oil. Mix in the onion for 5 minutes or until delicate. - Mix in the ginger and mustard seeds for 30 seconds or until sweet-smelling. Mix in the coconut for 1-2 minutes or until light and bright. Move to a bowl.

Put away to marginally cool. Mix in the tomato, bean stew, coriander, lime squeeze, and sugar.

-Preheat a grill barbecue or singe barbecue on high. Splash the fish with oil. Cook on the grill for 2-3 minutes on each side or until dazzling and fish pieces effectively when tried with a fork.

- Split the steamed vegetables amongst plates. Top with the fish and a teaspoon of the coconut mixture.

5. Veg Thai curry soup (Asian)

Ingredients:

1 bundle (8.8 ounces) scant rice noodles or uncooked holy messenger hair pasta.. 1 tablespoon sesame oil.. 2 tablespoons red curry glue.. 1 cup light coconut milk.. 1 container (32 ounces) of low sodium chicken stock.. or on the other hand veggie stock.. 1 tablespoon low sodium soy sauce or fish sauce.. 1 bundle (14

ounces) of firm tofu, depleted and diced.. 1 can (8-3/4 ounces) of full kid corn, depleted and cut down the center.. 1 can (5 ounces) of bamboo shoots, emptied 1-1/2 cups chopped young shiitake mushrooms.. 1/2 medium sweet red pepper, cut into slight strips. Torn new basil leaves and lime wedges

Method

- Plan noodles according to bundle bearings.
- In the meantime, in a 6-qt. stockpot, heat oil over medium intensity. Add curry glue; cook until aromatic, roughly 30 seconds. Slowly speed in coconut milk until blended. Mix in stock and soy sauce; heat to the point of boiling. Add tofu and vegetables to stockpot; simmer until vegetables are fresh and delicate, 3-5 minutes. Channel noodles; add to soup. Top each serving with basil; present with lime wedges.

6. Sugar Free panna cotta

Ingredients:

1 tablespoon gelatin 1 envelope.. 2 teaspoons cold water.. 2 cups heavy cream. 1 cup milk of option I utilized unsweetened coconut milk.. 1/3 cup granulated sugar of decision priest natural product sugar or erythritol.. 2 teaspoon vanilla concentration

Methods

- Delicately oil eight 1/2 cup or four 1 cup ramekins and put aside. In a tiny bowl, whisk together your gelatin with cold water. Allow it to sit to thicken.

In a pot, add your other fixings. On medium intensity, while mixing consistently, heat to the point of boiling. When it starts to boil, decrease it to incredibly low and let it stew for a few minutes, prior to removing it from the intensity.

- Add the gelatine blend into the pan and whisk well overall, until consolidated and smooth. - Convey the panna cotta combination among the ramekins and permit it to cool to room temperature. When cool, place them in the fridge for anything like 4 hours, or short-term.

- After the panna cotta has solidified, eliminate the panna cotta from the chiller. Utilizing a relatively moist blade, run it around the edges of the ramekin for quick evacuation. Flip around the ramekins onto a dish and serve.

Chapter 11: 5 Incredible Seeds for Blood Sugar Control

From methi seeds to sabja seeds, deal with your blood glucose levels with these astounding seeds that can also give flavor and fiber to your food.

There are sure seeds you may add to your cereals, smoothies, or bites that can keep you full for a really long time and check undesirable desires.

With regards to supervising diabetes, it is constantly recommended to add low GI food types to your eating routine that forestall abrupt sugar surges. Eating non-boring vegetables like broccoli, green verdant veggies, carrots, and natural goods like oranges, apples, berries, entire grains, and protein are critical elements of a sound diabetes diet as they contain the proper supplements and aid with further growing glucose resilience. How you create your food and what you add to your readiness can also add to the dietary benefit of a feast. Fenugreek seeds and ajwain seeds help in dialing back the assimilation of carbs and forestall sugar levels from abrupt shoots. Aside from that, there are sure seeds you may add to your grains, smoothies, or snacks that can keep you full for a great lengthy time and control unpleasant desires.

Urvashi Agarwal, Nutritionist, Integrative Wellbeing Mentor, and Hormonal Wellbeing

Expert recommends 5 seeds that can aid with managing diabetes.

1. Methi Seeds (Fenugreek Seeds):
The solvent fiber present in fenugreek seeds called "Galactomannan," is a crucial fixer that dials back the pace of processing and retention of carbs. Thus, this brings down blood glucose levels in diabetics and improves glucose resistance.

2. Ajwain Seeds (Carom Seeds):
They might be utilized to regulate diabetes in view of their substantial fiber content, which assists in settling glucose levels. Furthermore, the seeds contain mitigating and cell reinforcement effects, and they assist with quickening digestion. These benefits can encourage weight reduction, which is advantageous for supervising diabetes.

3. Sabja Seeds (Basil Seeds):
They contain a ton of fiber. In a few tests, diabetic patients were oftentimes supplied sabja seeds just before dinners, which forestalled the blood glucose flood. Sabja seeds were discovered as absolutely appealing in preserving glucose levels in persons with type 2 diabetes.

4. Also Seeds (Flax Seeds):
They are undoubtedly profitable for us. They contain heaps of insoluble fiber, which supports the body's glucose levels as well as deals with our stomach's well-being. As stated by a new investigation, flaxseeds have a better probability

of reducing the pervasiveness of type 1 as well as type 2 diabetes. This is a direct outcome of flax lignan found in them.

5. Kaddu Seeds (Pumpkin Seeds):

Loaded with intensifiers like Trigonelline (TRG), Nicotinic corrosive (NA), and D-chiro-inositol (DCI), pumpkin seeds are wonderful for diabetes patients. They additionally contain protein, dietary fiber, omega-6 fats, and magnesium which are actually fantastic for diabetes executives.

In this way, remember these seeds for your usual eating regimen to counter diabetes, and live contentedly.

Conclusion

As we wrap up our journey through the pages of "Mastering Diabetes: The Revolutionary Method to Reverse Insulin Resistance Permanently," it's not about reaching a finish line—it's about embracing a lifestyle shift. Picture this as a roadmap rather than a final destination. The revolutionary method we've explored isn't a one-size-fits-all remedy; it's a toolkit for you to mold and shape according to your unique journey with diabetes.

Think of it as a dance between your daily choices and the rhythm of your body. Dive into your kitchen, experimenting with the vibrant palette of foods that can nourish and empower. Lace-up your sneakers, not for a marathon, but for the joy of movement that speaks to your body's language. Unwind in the serenity of mindful moments and let the healing power of restful sleep envelop you like a warm hug.

This isn't a goodbye; it's an invitation to a continuous dialogue with your well-being. Embrace the little victories and learn from the detours. Seek support when the road feels rocky, and celebrate the sweetness of progress. As you step into the world armed with newfound knowledge and an empowered mindset, remember, you're not just managing diabetes; you're mastering the art of living well—unapologetically and vibrantly. Your journey continues, and the possibilities are as boundless as your commitment to your health.

Appendix

À. C-Peptide Testing:

If diabetes were a puzzle, C-peptide testing would be one of its elusive pieces, quietly influencing the picture of insulin production and offering insights into the intricacies of the body's metabolic dance. Let's embark on a journey into the realm of C-peptide testing, demystifying its significance and shedding light on its role in the diagnosis and management of diabetes.

What Is C-Peptide, Anyway?
At first glance, the term "C-peptide" might sound like a cryptic code from a medical manual. In reality, it's a small but mighty protein produced in the pancreas along with insulin. Think of insulin and C-peptide as inseparable dance partners – both born from the same precursor molecule. When insulin is released into the bloodstream, it brings C-peptide along

for the ride. So, why does this dynamic duo matter?

A Window into Insulin Production
C-peptide serves as a unique window into the world of insulin production. Unlike insulin, C-peptide doesn't get absorbed by the body's cells. It lingers in the bloodstream, offering a reliable measure of how much insulin the pancreas is producing. This makes C-peptide testing a valuable tool in distinguishing between natural insulin and synthetic insulin injected by those managing diabetes.

A Diagnostic Detective: C-Peptide Testing in Action
Imagine your body as a bustling city, and insulin as the traffic director ensuring the smooth flow of glucose. But what happens when this director goes on strike, leading to chaotic traffic jams of elevated blood sugar? C-peptide testing steps in as the detective, helping unravel the mystery of why the insulin-producing machinery may be malfunctioning.

Type 1 Diabetes: The Silent Clues

In the realm of Type 1 diabetes, C-peptide testing becomes a subtle detective, revealing the silent clues left by the immune system's assault on the insulin-producing beta cells. Low C-peptide levels in Type 1 diabetes signify a reduced capacity for the pancreas to produce insulin, shedding light on the autoimmune battle within.

Type 2 Diabetes: A Balancing Act

For those grappling with Type 2 diabetes, C-peptide testing becomes a measure of the delicate balancing act between insulin resistance and the pancreas's efforts to meet the body's demands. Elevated or normal C-peptide levels here tell a tale of resilience – the pancreas striving to keep pace with the insulin resistance posed by the body.

Prediabetes: A Whisper of Warning

In the shadowy realm of prediabetes, where blood sugar levels tiptoe into the danger zone, C-peptide testing becomes a whisper of warning. Elevated C-peptide levels might indicate the pancreas working overtime to compensate for the body's insulin resistance – a subtle signal that all may not be well on the metabolic front.

Gestational Diabetes: A Temporary Unveiling
In the unique landscape of gestational diabetes, where pregnancy introduces a complex interplay of hormones, C-peptide testing unveils the temporary adjustments made by the pancreas. Elevated C-peptide during pregnancy might signify a heightened insulin production, revealing the body's adaptation to the increased demand imposed by gestation.

Navigating Treatment Options
Armed with the insights gained from C-peptide testing, individuals and healthcare professionals can chart a course through the maze of treatment options. Whether it's adjusting insulin dosages, exploring lifestyle modifications, or considering

innovative therapies, the information gleaned from C-peptide testing becomes a compass guiding personalized care.

In the Grand Symphony of Diabetes
In the grand symphony of diabetes management, C-peptide testing emerges as a harmonious note, playing its part in orchestrating tailored strategies for individuals across the diabetes spectrum. It's not merely a diagnostic tool but a storyteller, narrating the tale of insulin production, resistance, and adaptation within the intricate tapestry of the human body.

So, the next time you encounter the term "C-peptide," envision it as a storyteller whispering the secrets of your body's insulin ballet – a vital element in the ongoing saga of mastering diabetes.

B. Green List of Diabetes-Friendly Foods

Embarking on a journey to manage diabetes involves more than just counting carbs; it's about embracing a lifestyle that nurtures your well-being. One key aspect is your food choices. We've compiled a comprehensive list of green list foods, each packed with goodness and suitable for keeping your blood sugar levels in check. Let's delve into a world of flavors and health!

1. Leafy Greens: The Heroes of the Plate

Kicking off our list are the champions of the green realm - leafy greens. Spinach, kale, collard greens, and lettuce are rich in fiber, vitamins, and antioxidants. Not only do they add vibrant color to your plate, but they also support stable blood sugar levels.

2. Cruciferous Crusaders

Broccoli, cauliflower, Brussels sprouts, and cabbage form the formidable lineup of cruciferous vegetables. These powerhouses are not only low in carbs but also boast anti-inflammatory properties, making them ideal for diabetes management.

3. The Allium Allies

Garlic, onions, leeks, and shallots are the allium wonders that bring a burst of flavor to your dishes. Beyond taste, they contribute to heart health and have blood sugar-regulating properties, making them a must-add to your green list.

4. Avocado: Nature's Butter

Creamy, delicious, and loaded with healthy fats, avocados are a diabetes-friendly delight. Packed with monounsaturated fats and fiber, they help control blood sugar and keep you feeling satisfied. Guacamole, anyone?

5. Berries: Nature's Sweet Treats

Strawberries, blueberries, raspberries, and blackberries are not just tasty; they're packed with antioxidants and fiber. These natural sweet treats add a splash of color to your diet without causing dramatic spikes in blood sugar.

6. Nuts and Seeds: Crunchy Goodness

Almonds, walnuts, chia seeds, and flaxseeds bring a satisfying crunch to your meals. Rich in healthy fats, fiber, and protein, they provide a steady release of energy, making them perfect for maintaining blood sugar stability.

7. Fatty Fish: Omega-3 Super Heroes

Rich supplies of omega-3 fatty acids can be found in salmon, mackerel, sardines, and trout. These healthy fats contribute to heart health and have anti-inflammatory properties, making them a wise choice for those managing diabetes.

8. Lean Proteins: Satisfying Sustenance

Chicken, turkey, tofu, and legumes provide a protein-packed punch without sending your blood sugar on a rollercoaster ride. Including lean proteins in your meals helps maintain energy levels and promotes satiety.

9. Whole Grains: The Fiber Force

Quinoa, brown rice, oats, and barley are whole grains that offer a steady release of energy. Packed with fiber, they help regulate blood sugar levels and keep you feeling full, making them a valuable addition to your green list.

10. Greek Yogurt: Probiotic Powerhouse

Rich in protein and probiotics, Greek yogurt supports gut health and helps control blood sugar levels. Choose plain, unsweetened varieties to avoid added sugars, and enjoy it as a satisfying snack or breakfast option.

11. Cinnamon: Spice with Benefits

Not just a flavor enhancer, cinnamon has been shown to improve insulin sensitivity. Sprinkle it on your morning oatmeal or add a dash to your coffee for a delicious and diabetes-friendly boost.

12. Green Tea: Sip Your Way to Health

Swap sugary drinks for the simplicity of green tea. Packed with antioxidants, it not only supports metabolism but also aids in managing blood sugar levels. Plus, it's a refreshing alternative to high-calorie beverages.

13. Tomatoes: Versatile and Vibrant

Tomatoes, whether fresh or in sauce form, bring a burst of color and flavor to your dishes. Rich in lycopene and vitamins, they add a nutritional punch to your meals. Opt for fresh tomatoes in salads or enjoy them in cooked dishes for a delightful culinary experience.

14. Asparagus: Spears of Goodness

Asparagus not only adds elegance to your plate but is also a diabetes-friendly vegetable. Low in carbs and high in fiber, it supports digestive health and contributes to steady blood sugar levels. Roast, grill, or sauté for a tasty side dish.

15. Sweet Potatoes: Nature's Candy

Sweet potatoes offer a natural sweetness along with a dose of fiber and vitamins. With a lower glycemic index compared to regular potatoes, they make a delicious and nutritious addition to your green list. Roast or mash them for a satisfying and colorful side dish.

16. Eggs: Protein Powerhouses

Eggs are a versatile and protein-packed option for breakfast, lunch, or dinner. They provide essential nutrients and are a great choice for maintaining stable blood sugar levels. Scramble them, boil them, or make a vegetable-packed omelet for a hearty meal.

17. Bell Peppers: Colorful Crunch

Add a rainbow of bell peppers to your green list for a crunchy and vitamin-rich experience. Whether you prefer them raw in salads or sautéed in a stir-fry, bell peppers contribute to a balanced and visually appealing diet.

18. Legumes: Fiber-Full Friends

Beans, lentils, and chickpeas are excellent sources of fiber and plant-based protein. Incorporating legumes into your meals not only helps control blood sugar levels but also provides long-lasting energy. Create hearty soups, stews, or salads for a satisfying meal.

19. Mushrooms: Umami Delights

Mushrooms bring a unique umami flavor to your dishes while being low in carbs and calories. They're versatile ingredients that can be grilled, sautéed, or added to soups and stews for a savory boost.

20. Dark Chocolate: Indulgence with Benefits

Yes, you read that right! Dark chocolate, in moderation, can be part of your green list. Choose varieties with higher cocoa content to enjoy the antioxidant benefits and a touch of sweetness without causing significant spikes in blood sugar.

Remember, the green list is about variety, balance, and enjoying your food. Feel free to experiment with different combinations, flavors, and cooking methods. Making choices that are diabetes-friendly doesn't have to mean compromising flavor—it just means appreciating the excitement of a colorful and nutritious culinary adventure. Explore the universe of foods on the green list, enjoy the tastes, and take pleasure in the benefits to your health. Both your health and your taste senses will appreciate it!